# Lecture Reprint Number 3

# How To Revitalize
# The Glands

by Bernard Jensen, D.C., N.D.,
Nutritionist

Revised and edited by Jon D. Jensen

## ACKNOWLEDGEMENTS

I acknowledge and give thanks to Betty Norlin for being such a wonderful friend and for continually encouraging me and assisting me on my book writing/editing journey. Author of *"Our Bodies: The Optimal Design."* www.bettynorlin.com www.whatisholistichealth.com

I acknowledge and give thanks to Daylin Anderson, B.S. in Psychology, Cognitive and Behavioral Neuroscience/Human Development, for editing and compiling information for this lecture reprint booklet series. Daylin is a cherished friend who typed up many of these booklets for me and made it possible to finish this project. She truly is my inspiration and muse.

I acknowledge and give thanks to Gary and Jeanne Nichols. They have given to me their expertise in editing and marketing as well as assisting me with my grandfather's videos taking them from video to DVD. They have always supported me whether it was creating an office space, writing, or giving lectures. Thank you both!

## COPYRIGHT

Copyright @ 2019 by Jon D. Jensen

Because of the dynamic nature of the Internet, any web addresses or links contained in this book may have changed since publication and may no longer be valid.

Paperback

ISBN-13: 978-1099770418

## DISCLAIMER

Any information given in this book is not intended to be taken as a replacement for medical advice. Any person with a condition requiring medical attention should consult a qualified health professional.

## INTRODUCTION

My name is Jon Jensen and I have been involved in the holistic health field for many years. I have published a nutrition book, "A Simple Guide to Healthy Living" as a way to communicate with people outside my client base with information I feel is key to a healthy life. It is available on Amazon or through my website, www.jensenholistichealth.com

I've wanted to publish these health booklets for many years. My intention for editing, revising, and publishing my grandfather's 21 lecture reprint booklets is rooted in my desire to continue his legacy of teaching right living through health and nutrition. Dr. Bernard Jensen spent his lifetime helping others to achieve health through education and his writing, and I feel strongly that the message is needed now more than ever.

I always marveled that my grandfather, Dr. Bernard Jensen, could write so many books and still travel, receive numerous awards, teach classes on Iridology, rejuvenation/regeneration, and tissue cleansing. These lecture reprints are the product of his first lectures, typed up and stapled into booklets and originally sold for ninety-nine cents each. Thus, the beginning of a pattern where he would write and self-publish many books over his lifetime. He did end up publishing books with a couple different publishing companies, but most of his work was self-published.

## DR. BERNARD JENSEN, PH.D., N.D., D.C.

One of the greatest healers the world has ever known. Dr. Bernard Jensen spent over 60 years as a pioneer in the holistic health field, helping to pave the way for the alternative health revolution that we are now experiencing.

Dr. Jensen began his career at the West Coast Chiropractic College where Bernard became the youngest chiropractor in the state of California. He traveled extensively in search of health knowledge, a search that led him to over 65 countries to observe the lifestyles of the people and their various ways of eating. Each place provided a different health secret.

Throughout his career, Dr. Jensen wrote and published over 60 books. After working with over 350,000 patients, Dr. Jensen firmly believed that nutrition is the greatest single therapy to be applied in the holistic healing arts and that "We must treat the patient, not just the disease."

Born on March 25, 1908, to parents of Danish descent, Eugen and Anna Jensen, Jorgen Bernard Jensen was raised in Stockton, California, then a small rural town in one of the richest agricultural valleys of the state. The unexpected death of his mother at age 29 from tuberculosis and consumption left three children to be raised by their father, Eugen Jensen, who was a chiropractor. Very little has been written about Bernard's early life growing up in Stockton, his brother and sister, and a few comments in lectures he made about his father who was mentioned as very strict and analytical.

Early in life, young Bernard displayed the qualities needed for his future work. His penchant for being an analytical, critical, serious perfectionist blended with his sensitive, competitive, spiritual-minded personality to arm him with an unusual perspective that opened the doors to the unconventional life he was soon to enter. But before that path was firmly set, several intense learning experiences occurred which determined the direction he was to take.

Being his own worst obstacle, restless and never satisfied, he would rather study and read a book than eat or sleep. His father was a chiropractor, and young Bernard followed in his path. When he was 18 years old, Bernard entered the West Coast Chiropractic College in Oakland, California. During his four years of study, Bernard burned the midnight oil while holding down as many as two outside jobs simultaneously. The strain was immense. The capacity to push forward and the ability to persevere doggedly toward a goal were firmly established, but there was a price to pay. Bernard supported himself by working at a dairy in his spare time, and the long hours of work and study, along with poor food habits, took a heavy toll on Bernard's health. After receiving his diploma in 1929, Dr. Bernard Jensen went into practice, opening his first office in Oakland, California. He focused intently on the task of his calling which was to offer a helping hand to those suffering and in need. Dr. Bernard Jensen's devotion was complete, the hours long, his personal needs forgotten. By this time, the sacrificing of many years began to demand attention. His health began to fail. A Medical Doctor diagnosed his condition as bronchiectasis, an often-fatal lung condition, with no known cure at the time. "There is nothing I can do for you," he was told.

The young man refused to give up, searching out a Seventh Day Adventist Medical Doctor who taught him basic nutritional principles, told Dr. Bernard Jensen to leave junk food alone and promptly presented him with a maintenance program involving natural health that emphasized the return to a pure, natural, and whole foods regimen. Following this program brought excellent results. Dr. Bernard Jensen was soon on the way back to health and renewed vitality. A great turning point had occurred. To be able to study nutrition and discover the laws of right living became his burning desire. Dr. Bernard Jensen turned the experience of what he learned from the Seventh Day Adventist Medical Doctor about the holistic approach into helping his patients get better and teaching them how to prevent themselves from getting sick. Dr. Bernard Jensen began taking breathing exercises with Thomas Gaines, once an instructor for the New York City Police Department. Slowly, and over a period of time, his health returned, and his lungs eventually healed completely.

Using this knowledge in working with his patients the results were dramatic and effective. Dr. Bernard Jensen's attention was now riveted in this direction. Natural therapeutics became his healing mode, setting the pattern for the rest of his life. He began to travel in search of more knowledge and information.

After Dr. Bernard Jensen opened his first office in Oakland, California, in 1929, he later moved to Los Angeles and expanded his practice to include branch offices at Long Beach and Santa Monica, with several chiropractors working under him. Such success had not come about overnight. In Chicago, Dr. Bernard Jensen took his post-graduate work at the National Chiropractic College and later from the Los Angeles Chiropractic College closer to home. Upon returning to California, he began an intensive study and investigation of something he was recently just learning about, the subject of iridology.

Dr. Bernard Jensen used Rocine's work as the basis for the programs used in his sanitariums—first a 25-bed sanitarium in San Leandro, California, then others in Ben Lomand and Alta Dena, and finally an 85-bed sanitarium at hidden Valley Health Ranch in Escondido, California. The sanitariums were quite successful, demonstrating the effectiveness of Rocine's ideas in working with patients. It was the Hidden Valley Health Ranch in Escondido that provided the greatest opportunity for applying the rules of right living. People in search of health and rejuvenation came to the ranch from all over the world to learn the principles that Dr. Bernard Jensen believed in, practiced, and taught.

Proper nutrition, together with sunshine, rest, exercise, fresh air, and positive attitudes helped thousands of patients at Dr. Bernard Jensen's sanitariums leave behind the symptoms of chronic diseases that they had developed.

Patients came from all over the world, some to stay at his sanitariums, others for outpatient consultations, and still others to attend his classes in rejuvenation and Food Studies. Thousands of New Zealanders formed clubs to follow his dietetic advice, filling out the over 350,000 people he reached, accumulated over the years. He acquired a multitude of experiences from these people individually and in group studies, acquiring information and summing it up for use in his healing work and writing.

Dr. Bernard Jensen visited the Hunza Valley, where disease, doctors, dentists, and hospitals were practically nonexistent and where there were no jails, prisons or police, because there was no crime. One of Dr. Bernard Jensen's highlights of that trip was staying as a guest of the Mir of Hunza's palace for 10 days.

Dr. Bernard Jensen visited the Caucasus Mountains in the USSR to meet a 153-year-old man who had stopped riding horseback a few years earlier only because of his doctor's orders. Dr. Bernard Jensen traveled to Vilacamba, Ecuador, where heart patients were able to recuperate so marvelously. Everywhere Dr. Bernard Jensen went, he brought back some new remedy or approach to integrate into the system he taught his patients.

Dr. Bernard Jensen received his Ph.D. at the age of 75 from the University of Humanistic Studies, San Diego, California.

Dr. Bernard Jensen retired from active chiropractic practice in 1978, and devoted himself to teaching, writing, and lecturing on the subjects of nutrition, rejuvenation, and iridology. Around this time, Dr. Bernard Jensen completed work on a two-hour feature film, titled "World Search for Health,

Happiness and Long Life," narrated by actor Dennis Weaver.

The Academy of Science in Paris awarded Dr. Bernard Jensen a medal in 1971 for exceptional services rendered to humanity. Also, in the same year, 1971, Dr. Bernard Jensen received an honorary doctorate from the Center for the Study of Human Sciences in Lisbon, Portugal.

At a ceremony in San Remo, Italy in 1973, Dr. Bernard Jensen was presented the Ignatz Von Peczely International Iridology Gold Medal by the World Congress of Scientific Medicine, an organization embracing many medical and health disciplines.

A congress of health professionals at Aixen Provence, France, in 1974, recognized Dr. Bernard Jensen with an award for his "valuable contribution in the field of iridology."

Then in 1975, the International Naturopathic Association honored Dr. Bernard Jensen for his service to mankind through his work in the fields of health, Iridology, and nutrition.

Knighted into the Order of St. John of Malta in 1978 for his humanitarian work in the field of health, Dr. Bernard Jensen was awarded the cross of St. John at a special ceremony in New York City. This Order is the oldest chivalric organization in the world, tracing its origin back to the time preceding the first Crusade.

In 1981, at the Fifth Annual Herb Symposium, the Agnes Arber Distinguished Service award was presented to Dr. Bernard Jensen for his contributions to the current "herb renaissance."

In 1982, the National Health Federation honored Dr. Bernard Jensen with its Pioneer Doctor of the Year award at its annual convention in Long Beach, California.

In 1982, Dr. Bernard Jensen traveled to Brussels, Belgium to accept the 1982 Dag Hammarskjold award of the Pax Mundi Academy, an international organization which presents annual awards to those in the arts and sciences who have made outstanding contributions in their fields. The award, in the category of scientific merit, was for "the exceptional services rendered to collective humanity... toward international cooperation and solidarity..." Dr. Bernard Jensen was personally congratulated on his award by U. S. Ambassador, Charles Price.

In 1988 Dr. Bernard Jensen held his 80th Birthday Celebration at the Town and Country Hotel in San Diego, California, where people came from all over the world to celebrate his 80 years of life and work in the holistic health field.

In 1993 he was presented with a PhD. in natural healing arts and sciences from Westbrook University, where his iridology course was part of the school curriculum.

In 1998 and 1999 Dr. Bernard Jensen received awards from the IIPA for his work in iridology.

In 2000 Dr. Bernard Jensen was awarded by Nature Sunshine an honorary award for his outstanding contributions to iridology and herbology before five thousand people.

On February 22, 2001 a month before his 93$^{rd}$ birthday, Dr. Bernard Jensen passed away at 92 years old.

The short biography above about Dr. Bernard Jensen is a small part of a larger biography I am writing about my grandfather's life. If you are interested in learning more I will be blogging and have more information at www.bernardjensen.org.

In the 21 lecture reprint booklets you'll see products or foods that might not be commonly found today. I left some things in to give the flavor of that time period and what he was thinking at that time. I also left in quotes or sayings from that era. I edited misspellings and grammatical errors. Overall, I feel that these booklets give down to earth advice and can still be regarded as basic knowledge in the mainstream health field today. A lot of his products are no longer available, but you can find what remains on my website, www.jensenholistichealth.com.

I hope you enjoy these lecture reprint booklets as much as I do and take them for what they are. If nothing else, a novelty and glimpse of the past. A simple approach from one of the early promoters of healthy living. Alongside such greats of that era like Paul Bragg, Jack LaLanne, Dr. Max Gerson, V.E. Irons, and Dr. Bronner at the beginning of a health revolution.

Jon D. Jensen

# HOW TO REVITALIZE THE GLANDS

*"My purpose is to serve and I must serve my purpose."*

## Bernard Jensen, Ph.D., D.C., N.D.

## REVITALIZE YOUR GLANDS

In dealing with the subject of glands today, we are just dealing with the glands in which most people are interested. When we talk about glands, the average person thinks of the glands that control our weight; glands that control our sexual life and the glands that have to do with most of the doctors' treatments that we hear discussed or have heard of through advertisements in the paper and over the radio.

It is well to take inventory as we go through life to find out what is behind the cause. There is a cause behind every case and when we see a condition developing we must get to the initial cause.

For instance: A man came into my office and said, "you told my wife that my child did not need to have her tonsils taken out. I took my little girl to another doctor and he says they should be taken out immediately. Who am I going to believe?" I advised him to believe whatever he wished to, but at least he should try the advice of the person who said the operation was unnecessary because after the tonsils are taken out, it would be too late to do any corrective work. I asked him to call the doctor and find out what, in the doctor's opinion, was causing the trouble in the tonsils. The doctor told him that it could be stomach trouble. I asked, "well, why didn't you ask him what is causing the stomach trouble?" When he called the doctor again, the doctor stated that it could be the child's diet that was causing the stomach trouble. I said, "Well, why not start cutting out the kind of a diet that is causing a bad stomach, that in turn may be causing the bad tonsils. That is where I begin."

There are causes behind the cause, and I am interested in getting to first causes. I am not interested in helping anyone stimulate the glands or make just the glandular life work.

You have heard of the stomach operations in which young vital glands are transplanted into the body. What are you going to do with good, young-working glands in an old body? These are not going to stay young and are going to tear the old body to pieces. You will find you are going to have young ideas, but no way to follow through on these ideas. You are going to be able to accomplish things as far as the glands are concerned, but you will find out that you haven't the body to go with it.

I think that if you are going to have young glands, you should have a young body to go with them, and a young mind to make them all work. So, it must be a matter of complete rejuvenation, physically, mentally, and spiritually, in order to get all the good you should have.

When you hear about the stomach operations for the rejuvenation of the body through gland transplantation, you are not told of the thousands of transplantations of glands that were done on human bodies before there was one that proved successful. You have only heard of the successful ones. Thousands have gone through this transplantation of glands in the body, but there are very few successes.

There are certain secrets that we have to discover before we can develop a good glandular system. We know that a good glandular system will come only when we do first things first. The first thing is the realization that our body, in all of its physical expressions, does not know what to do until it has been given the stimulus from another center, and this is the mind and the spirit. The finger cannot move of its own accord to accomplish something, unless the accomplishment and the goal and the attainment is in the mind first. The physical body does not know what to do. The physical body follows; it does not lead.

This I want you to recognize, when we deal with the glands. So many people are interested in working with the glands as a cause of trouble, and after all, they are an effect. The glands will move just like your finger will move when the goal and the attainment are right.

Most of us are looking for hormones or other kinds of stimulation to the glands, when after all, we have all that we need situated in our own body. This stimulation, however, needs to be cared for and nourished in other centers of our body. Inspiration and aspiration and loving kindness will do more for the glands than anything else, while cruelty, hatred, fear, envy, and jealousy will dry up the glands. A poverty consciousness will squeeze glands dry. We find that our glands follow our mental attitude, just as our fingers do, or just as we arise from a chair. If you have the inspiration to get out of a chair to accomplish something, it is done entirely different than if there is nothing to look forward to. In other words, many times we will stay in the chair just because we have no reason to rise. Our whole physical body reacts in the same way, whether it be the fingers or the muscles, the liver, the stomach, or the glands.

The association of ideas is very powerful. I was telling a man at one time about apples and how good they were, and he said, "Don't talk about apples to me." I asked, "Why not?" he said, "Well, you know, at one time I fell out of an apple tree and broke my arm. I landed in a hospital and I married my nurse. I've been in a heck of a fix ever since!" We have this association of ideas. Every time he sees an apple, he doesn't want to even think of it because it got him into a marriage in which he was unhappy.

Too many people today are expecting some muscle rejuvenation program to give them a good body. You are an empty shell, and the good we can accomplish comes from within. The way we fill this shell for ourselves is by starting from the inside with our good building work and allowing the outside changes to follow. My work is not trying to find a way to make a new body from capsules, pills, or an operation. After all, the rejuvenation comes in the mind, and it is necessary to be "transformed in mind and spirit." This mental and spiritual transformation starts rejuvenation in the physical body and we find that the body follows right along in its rejuvenation.

Gracious gesture, we must first have the gracious gesture in mind. To walk graciously, we must have the mind so coordinated with the physical body that all that we do physically is walk graciously. Many people may have a dance in their heads, but unless practiced and worked out in expression, the dance cannot be performed.

There are so many today who are expecting a happy marriage as soon as they can have a better stomach, as soon as they can have better food, as soon as the physical things have changed. So many people are complaining about their wives or complaining about their husbands.

If we are forced through inharmonious circumstances to develop a program of resentment or resistance in our bodies we begin to push the things away that may be the dearest things in our lives to us. So the first thing we must do is be transformed in our minds and in our spirit. The hand, the body, the muscles you tense, the sexual organs, the glands (the thyroid gland and pituitary particularly), every organ and gland in your body responds to the thoughts you think.

To get a love reaction from the glands in the body we have to recognize this one point first: There is no love reaction in the glands until there is love in the mind. Your glands respond to what is in the mind. You cannot make the organs do things unless it is first done in the mind. This is probably the hardest thing for you to see, but you must try to recognize this fact. Let us see what the body can teach us; let us learn a few of the fundamentals; and then let us see what can happen to the different organs through our thought processes and the way we live.

Do you know that men and women are exactly alike in structure? Did you know that the organs a woman has, a man has? It may surprise you when I say that men and women have to be treated alike because their minds function alike. Women need love. Men need love. And there are women who make just as fierce fighters as men can be. Just because a woman is a woman does not mean she has to be treated any more dearly than a man does. This is something to think about isn't it?

I know some men who have to be treated like China dolls or they break easily. And some women you have to talk rough to...they are built that way. That is the way mental temperament is. . .it is apart from the glandular system. When we speak of this glandular system or about these mental processes, let us first see where life comes from. The life more abundant that has been promised to you, must be seen through your inner sight first. You cannot have the life more abundant merely through foods or a doctor's treatment . . .or from some glandular stimulant. What is the use of having the glands in good working order and not having the love channels developed? If you develop the love channels then the glands will respond. So start first with the mind.

In speaking of the difference between man and woman, I might say that there are cases where the woman has changed into a man. There are even medical records where men have given birth to babies. In this last war a Russian general walked into a hospital. His sex had changed so much in a few years that he had a baby. It has been recorded in Los Angeles a short time ago that a woman changed into a man. Did you know that in the Olympic Games they make sure now that all women have a complete physical examination because many of the women who have been wonderful athletes, wonderful runners, wonderful javelin throwers, have changed from one sex to the other? Mary Weston who appeared in the Olympic Games and took all the records for women finally changed to a man. Her name is now Mark Weston, instead of Mary Weston.

I repeat, the organs in men and women are exactly the same. They may be in different positions or a different size, but I am bringing this point out to show you that both the male and female organs do the same work as far as expression is concerned. In their development they need the same care, the same outlook, the same spirit, the same kind of thinking. It is not a matter of the glands themselves or the relation between the man and the woman. It is the relation between the mind and the glands. Set your mind right first. Put your own house in order and you will find the best will come to you. So many people say, "It was his fault." Maybe it was your fault. But as far as faults are concerned it is probably just a lack of understanding. There are really no faults, except in our own thinking.

In looking at the glands, we start from the top of the head first. The pituitary gland is found in the head, right behind the nose. This is the master gland in the body. The pituitary gland controls the weight, you've seen a lot of women who have what is called a pituitary apron, or a heavy fat apron hanging in the lower abdomen. It just seems to be an excess amount of fat. Men can have this too. It controls our femininity, our masculinity. You have seen a lot of women who are very masculine. And you have seen a lot of men who are feminine. We find it depends on their inheritance. A man can inherit the masculine characteristics of the father, depending upon the inherent aim that they have taken onto themselves.

The pituitary gland controls the bones in the body. We find that dwarfs and huge giants are controlled by the pituitary gland. Hair follicles in the body are controlled by the pituitary gland. A woman can grow a mustache because of an unbalanced pituitary gland. A heavy hair growth on the legs of a woman can come from the pituitary gland. The pituitary gland is the master gland and controls femininity and masculinity and makes the difference between the two. This master gland also controls the thyroid. When the thyroid overworks, then the pituitary balances it by underworking. We know also that it is a master gland as far as the ovaries are concerned, where the orchic glands are concerned and the prostate gland. All of these glands must have a balancer, which is the pituitary gland as its work is to balance all the other glands in the body.

The pineal gland in the brain is called the sixth sense gland. There is very little known about this gland but it is claimed to be the psychic gland, or the third eye. There are many names for this gland. You cannot exactly say it is a sex gland, but these glands are so interrelated, one with the other, that it is difficult to say that this gland or the other is the sex gland. Some people have an idea you have one or two glands in your body and that these two glands control all sex. This is a misapprehension as your liver also controls your sex. Your kidneys, your blood stream, your thyroid gland and the pituitary gland all play a part in your sex control. The pituitary gland, as we have already stated, controls almost everything in the body. Every gland in your body is related to the nervous system also, and the nervous system and the glandular system are in many ways alike in their activity and chemical makeup.

In regard to the pineal gland, we find that more has been said about this particular gland in our occult studies than in our physical studies. There is very little known about this gland from a physical standpoint.

When the Good Lord put our body together he made everything for a purpose, and you can readily see that everything is so interrelated that we cannot do without any one part. There are a lot of unseen things working in our body in functional form. This body is an organic accomplishment that man will never know all about. For that reason, we will never know everything there is to know about all the glands or any one gland in particular.

The pineal gland has a lot to do with the tie between people. I do believe that mental telepathy and a lot of our psychic influences in the world are handled in the pineal gland. That is the reason why so many people have considered it the psychic gland. When the pineal gland is well developed, we have good feelings toward one another, or no feelings at all. We learn from our occult studies much of the thread that binds people is found in the pineal gland. We are sensitive to another person's actions through the pineal gland.

We say that many of these glands are in our body for self-preservation, we mean they also take a part in our mental activity. Many people come to us who are married and feel very insecure. Where would you operate to find the security organ? Where would the surgeon operate to eliminate insecurity in life? There are many women who do not want money but want security. They have a feeling of loneliness, depression, and of being lost in this world. They have a feeling they will not be cared for in the future. We find that the tie between the man and the woman is not complete and their love for one another is incomplete. This tie is found more probably in the pineal gland than we realize.

I believe that the location of the glands in the body has a lot to do with their spiritual use. We find that man begins to live the physical life in his very early years; in the middle of his life, he lives the mental life, and the last part of his life he reaches out for the spiritual things. We find that the sexual organs are placed in the lower part of the body and it seems that sex is the one ultimate thought, ultimate gain, and the desire of those who are young. To overcome these lower thoughts and of the lower organs, we find that ultimately we raise our thoughts to the higher glands. Most of us in the mental world are just halfway there. We are situated in this metaphysical world, much as the thyroid gland is situated in our body, about halfway. In this world of so many religious changes, financial changes, and commercial changes, we are really a race of thyroid disturbances today.

Those people who can rise above the strife of the world today, have to reach for higher thoughts and the higher things. We find the pituitary and the pineal gland that are found in the head represent the highest thoughts possible. I do believe they respond to the more spiritual things.

When you start feeding the glands, you also feed the nerves. If you break down the nervous system, you also break down the glands. You cannot have a broken down nervous system and a good glandular system. When you break down one part of your body, the entire body goes with it. If you have a toxic body from a poor liver condition, then all the glands are toxic also and toxic glands cannot do good work.

If you recognize this as a truth, then you will realize what it is to a gland specialist or to treat one part of the body only. We cannot treat just one part of the body.

When we recognize that the glands are fed by the bloodstream and to treat one gland, and not the bloodstream, is not treating the cause; we then realize we are only treating an effect. It is like having an operation for some growth in the body, or some condition which has been built there by the blood. You cannot operate and take out the blood. When we treat the body, we should treat the whole body. We should recognize the body as a physical, mental, and spiritual book, and as we unfold its problems we must look at it in all three directions. It is impossible to have a good body physically and have a poor mind. There are elements in the mind that are just as necessary to care for as elements of the physical body.

When we speak of the sex glands, I want you to recognize that there is nothing crude or bad about sex. Some people put a filthy side to sex, but there is a beautiful side to sex also. Sex, if it is beautiful, means the glands are right, and all things that you do are done beautifully. The person who is well balanced sexually...I am talking about the glands. . .has every expression in every direction in beauty. There is nothing so beautiful as any Godly expression. So, it is all one, and has to be looked at as beautiful. I am not interested here now in just rejuvenating the sex glands to be used without having a beautiful expression of mind. This must go hand in hand or you will be running after vitamins and gland stimulants to try to build up the glands, if you do not take care of the rest of your body. . .and particularly the mind.

I mentioned how the pituitary gland shows certain reactions in the body. The pituitary gland also shows other relations, for when you overwork, the nervous system and the pituitary gland are unable to take the heavy load and this is reflected mentally. It will produce a very shiny top to the forehead and the skin will become very tight. When I look at a person, I can immediately tell the balance of his glands. This is just one of the little secrets I use.

It is easy to tell the pituitary balance in the body by looking at the forehead. Sometimes I can look at a person and see that he has one type of skin and just as it comes to the top of the forehead the skin changes and shows a definite tightness. I can tell then that the mental relation and the pituitary gland is breaking down. There may be wrong thoughts in the mind regarding the different glands in the body and the pituitary gland will feel this as you are a bundle of feelings. Every gland is a bundle of feelings. . . you feel with your glands, your personality is in your glands, you smile with your glands. That is why most of us do not smile enough; our glands are not good enough. Our smile and our glands work together.

It is claimed that your personality comes from your glands, and this is true. We have the chicken and the egg story. You cannot tell me which is first. You cannot have chickens without eggs and you cannot have eggs without chickens. So we must have had a start and the start was before either one. So we have to look to that start for our wonderful inspiration and for the beginning of all activity in our body, whether it be mind, glands, or the physical body.

In working with the body, whether diagnosing or treating, we realize that we must look at the body as a threefold organism. We must look to all the physical things that can be wrong—mental wrongs—and spiritual wrongs—and then in the treatment we must look in these three different directions. It matters not whether we start the treatment of a case mentally, physically, or spiritually. These three are all so interrelated, as you will see, that you may start mentally with your patient, or you may start physically. We do only one third of the job if we work in only one direction and do not consider the other.

I once saw a very small lady lift a piano off a child. A man could not have lifted that piano alone. But when the time came that she had to do it, she did it. Another instance of this kind was a lady who had been in a wheelchair for fourteen years and was living alone in Long Beach when they had an earthquake. She got out of that wheelchair and moved. There is nothing that will keep you standing still if you have the spirit first. Spirit is the motivating power. I also saw a lady's hair change from black to grey in less than ten minutes in the earthquake in Long Beach. What is it that feels all these things? When you walk out in the street and a horn is blown, do you stand still or do you jump out of the way? It depends on how the adrenal glands, which is one of the glands that feel, are performing. The adrenal glands are found right above the kidneys. They really feel!

There are reactions set up in the body upon receipt of a shock, a good or a bad telegram. We find that our body feels grief, even can be struck down by grief, but our glands feel and respond to the feelings first. These shock hormones get into the bloodstream in a hundredth part of a second in cases of accidents and shock, so that our body can respond immediately for its protection and preservation.

There are also glands that catch fear. They seem to be the seat of the instincts that protect us. These glands are subject to how we think, so it is very important that we do not have too much fear gripping the adrenal or thyroid gland. We start breaking down the adrenal and thyroid glands when we continually squeeze them too much. The hormones that are produced by the adrenal and thyroid and thrown into the bloodstream are so stimulated with that gland material that the heart goes faster, circulation is better, strength comes quickly and this is when we do the very unusual things just mentioned.

We find that extreme stimulation will bring on depression, an underactivity of the glands. You cannot stimulate a gland for any length of time, but what it is going to compensate and underact. Then, what do we have? A person has hay fever, asthmatic attacks, and we give them adrenalin! Is it possible that the gland has something to do with asthma? I am only trying to show you that when a person has an asthmatic attack, they inject adrenalin into the bloodstream. The adrenal gland has to be stimulated. An asthma attack comes when there has been an underactivity of that adrenal gland. This all affects the heart activity and heart work. Something for us to think about!

In discussing these different glands, I will show you the relationship between the glands and the diseases in your body. There is no disease that develops in your body but what every gland that I have mentioned has not some effect on it.

The thyroid gland is found at the base of the throat. Personally, I believe that the thyroid gland is the most abused gland in your body. Anatomically speaking, it is about the size of an almond, one on each side of the throat and very close together. Let us see how the thyroid gland controls the rest of the body. It controls the steadiness of the hands. We can tell that a person has a bad thyroid condition if his hands are shaking when he holds them in front of him.

Skin disturbances can be produced through the thyroid gland. We know that the temperature in our body is controlled by the thyroid gland. We know that waste is eliminated and broken down in the body by the thyroid gland. Do you see how necessary it is to have a good thyroid gland? And then think how we would mutilate it and break it down and expect our body to function properly. Well, don't you think we owe our body a good life? But where is the life? Most of us are trying to squeeze it out of the body, but after all, life is already set and we must live it. The thyroid gland also controls the calcium in the body. You cannot have tone, the energy, and the power to go on well if the thyroid glands are in an unbalanced condition.

Malfunction of every organ in the body, even overactivity, can come from the thyroid gland. Malnourishment can be caused by a poor thyroid gland; yet that thyroid only needs 1/1400 of a grain of Iodine daily. You can scarcely see that amount, yet, that is all that is needed daily to keep the thyroid gland physically well. We would not have to worry about running after gland foods if we did not wear out these elements faster than it is possible to replace them from our normal eating.

The thyroid gland, like the adrenal gland, is the gland of feeling, but it can also be called the watch dog. It filters your philosophy, if you have one. The person who does not know anything, cannot possibly be frightened, that person has no fears and no troubles, but just as soon as he has a little knowledge, at that moment he begins to qualify things. You say this is wrong, or that is right; I do not like this; I don't like that. The first thing you know, your thyroid gland gets tense from this very discrimination because you are not in good activity or pleasant surroundings; you are not in a peaceful atmosphere. You are inharmonious, in chaos, and the thyroid gland is trying its hardest to balance things. The thyroid gland is the gland that puts the brakes on your thinking. You have seen people with these huge eyes; the eyeballs seem to be protruding. This is a hyper-thyroid person. These people are working the thyroid gland too much.

There is a hormone produced by the thyroid gland called thyroxin. Thyroxin is a hormone that is necessary to take care of the nerve acids we develop in the body. Whenever we produce an excessive amount of nerve acids, the thyroxin takes over and balances these nerve acids. If you do not have enough thyroxin the thyroid gland has to work harder. When the thyroid gland works harder, more of these hormones are thrown into the bloodstream and we find we are better able to care for these excess nerve acids.

Some people do not know what it is to live normally mentally, and they wear out the thyroid gland so much that they produce goiters. Is it possible that we can produce a disease through our thinking? Watch the relation the glands have to our emotions. The thyroid gland tightens or relaxes our emotions.

I was asked whether bloodless surgery could help an enlarged thyroid. Bloodless surgery is a mechanical art, working with soft tissues in the body, and all it can do is to allow better flow of blood to these tissues. We can expect rejuvenation when we have more blood there, if it is good blood. Bloodless surgery can help tremendously in breaking down adhesions; allowing for greater circulation of blood in the lymph glands and in the muscle structure surrounding the thyroid gland. As far as a cure is concerned, however, there is nothing outside of what your own body can change to. There is no man who can put his hand on you and cure you. The cure comes from you and what you respond to. We find that all a doctor can do is remove obstructions, and then it is up to your body to come back to normal.

When a sanitarium patient of ours saw his blood count go up one million, five hundred thousand in one month's time, he said: "Why you are a miracle man!" Well, I could have administered the same treatment to a dead man and would have accomplished no results at all.

All I am, is an aid, a "first aid student to nature." I want to see perfect blood circulate in the body, and if there is anything obstructing it, like a man standing on the hose in the garden, I would like to get the foot off that hose so that a perfect stream of water can come through. And a perfect stream of blood should go to every organ of your body. If there are pressure symptoms, we remove them and after that, you and God work it out.

I was called to San Francisco on a case in which a young girl had developed a goiter. This girl's mother had told her she could not go around with a certain boyfriend, in school, and had kept her at home. The girl became so upset mentally that she was pining her life away. This was reflected on the thyroid gland so much that in six months a goiter was produced. I suggested that there was only one thing to do and that was to allow the girl to see her boyfriend. Surprisingly enough, after she had gone with this boyfriend for a certain length of time, the goiter disappeared.

Just to bring out what could be done in this particular case, we know that in feeding the thyroid gland, Iodine is very necessary. In most cases, according to our training, we should have fed this girl dulce tablets or Iodine in some way that would feed the gland physically. This was not enough, however, in this particular case, for this girl was wearing out the gland faster than we could possibly build it up with any food that we could give her.

In changing the mental attitude, the situation, the world in which these people were living, we were able to restore a normal condition.

You cannot say there is any one thing that does the work for the glands; there is a chemical story, a mental story, a story of circulation, a toxic story, and there is a right living story. You cannot just have an operation and say that is the cure. The cure is found only in right living. If you see the value of this work of right living, then you must recognize that right living is the only thing that can balance the body perfectly so that the ultimate of good health can be attained.

The thyroid gland is one of the glands that controls our grey or black hair. When you have a brittle condition of the hair we know that you lack Iodine or silicon. We know that you have been thinking too hard, that your philosophy is wrong. We know that the spiritual attitude of your life is not right. Is it not a surprising thing to say that we can feel your spiritual attitude in your hair? If it is through your thinking that you are breaking down the Iodine in your body, we realize that you should get Iodine back into the body, but above all things, don't you think you should get your thinking straightened out?

If a person developed a goiter in his younger life through eating the wrong foods and a lack of Iodine and then that person becomes more spiritually attuned, and yet the goiter hangs on through the change of diet and spiritual things, what can we expect or do in these cases?

Well, I might say that sometimes an organ has enlarged and has been stretched and strained to such an extent, it is almost impossible for the organ to go back into a normal shape again. In cases of varicose veins we sometimes find them enlarged to such extremes that it is very difficult for the veins to be brought back to a normal shape again. Sometimes, when we have straightened out our life physically, mentally, and spiritually, we find that a basal metabolism will show that the glands are doing all the work they are capable of doing with the thyroid gland, and that there is nothing more to be done, and the slight growth will just have to be endured. There may be a slight misshapen condition of the body, but unless that misshapen condition goes to the mind, I would leave it alone.

The average doctor today is living on the ignorance and the fears of the patient. We cannot have these fears operated on. I have seen many of these cases made much worse after an operation. If they would leave the condition to nature, they would live a longer and more normal life.

A short time ago, my wife and I were at Niagara Falls. This is a beautiful spectacle, two hundred feet high, and to see this huge amount of water going over this great drop and to think of ever being swept over the top of that, almost paralyzes one for a moment. There was a barge being towed by a ship and the cable suddenly broke. Two men were on this sand barge and they started floating toward the top of Niagara Falls, which meant they were going over the top of the Falls to certain death below. Do you know that one man's hair turned from black to grey in the twelve minutes that the barge was floating down toward the top of the Falls. This is how fear can grip a man and change his physical body. The thyroid gland and adrenal gland just froze this man. That is what you can do to your glands through your thinking. Not only that, but the other man died in a very few minutes. He killed himself by fear in a matter of minutes.

We are doing the same thing, only we do it more slowly. We are killing ourselves through a slow suicide process. We do not take care of ourselves properly through our thinking. I am only bringing this out because the physical things, the food ideas, the exercise they give you, is all so easy, so cut and dried, but I want you to see that the *most* important thing is the mind. If you do not get the mind straightened out you are going to be a doctor shopper; you are going to be constantly running after something to get yourself well. You cannot be well until the mind is straightened out, until the spirit is in a peaceful home. And I mean that sincerely.

There have been experiments made on the thyroid gland to ascertain its reactions. We know of a man in college who, during a freshman party, had his foot placed in a bucket. They blindfolded him, made a little scratch on his leg, and though there actually was no bleeding, they ran a little warm water down his leg from the scratch. When the water reached a point halfway up his leg, the man fainted! He believed the warm water was blood and was sure he was bleeding to death!

You can have joy in life or you can have depression. You can have anything you want in life. You can bring your glands to normal through your sight, or through how you accept the words you live by. You either live by the word of fear (fear killed a person every second and a half last year) or you live by the word of God. In nothing be anxious, "A merry heart doeth good like medicine." These are feelings my friends. If you cannot find these things you cannot have good glands.

In dealing with the body, whether it be mentally, physically, or spiritually, we recognize that the body works in this way: First, there is the thought in life; the thought is the first thing we have. This thought is either in good feeling or in bad feeling and we qualify this thought as it comes to us. We qualify inspirations, feelings, visions, and dreams that come to us. We even qualify the effects that foods may have on us. All thoughts that come to our mind are what we have to deal with first. Through every thought there is a sensation set up in the body.

These thoughts can be demonstrated in many ways. Just like I told you about the college student with his foot in the bucket. When he felt that hot water coming down his leg, he felt like it was filling up with blood and the thought of it produced a fainting spell. Now, you can suggest moonlight, a bench, and a park to a young boy and immediately you will find that a blush begins to develop; his cheeks will begin to get red. How did that blood come there? The thought produced the sensation and the next thing that happened was the expression. The expression is the thing that you see in the physical body. Behind every expression there first was the thought, then the sensation preceded the expression in the body. When the right thing comes first, we can expect a better expression. Attitude precedes every expression in the body.

A person who has a disorderly imagination has a disorderly glandular system as he is tense and it is working on his nervous system. Nine times out of ten, people who are frustrated have a disorderly imagination, the images before them are bad. They cannot qualify things around them and most of the things that are happening in the world in which they live are doing them harm. They are living under tension and fire. They are living under shrinking, striking, hatred, and chaos. These are reflected directly to the glands and what are they going to do? They can only reflect a poor expression toward life. Friction must be taken out of our life as we cannot live by or with friction. Where there is friction there is a misfit condition and the gears and wheels of life are not turning properly. They may need oil, soothing influences, but this should be taken care of as soon as possible. Irritation should be taken out. These are the things that wear out the glands more than anything else.

Glands are found in your feeling body and as long as we go through life feeling good, glands can usually be depended on to serve us well. If we are living a highly nervous life, a frustrated life, a life of personality disagreement, either with ourselves, our job, our wife, our family, our neighbors, or the world in general, we find out that we are in trouble.

Greed is something that will cause a great deal of trouble. Being a penny pincher will pinch every gland in your body and squeeze all the good out of them.

There is no home in which finances should be discussed if there is going to be resistance in the talking about them. I know there are many homes where money is a paramount issue. There are money problems and they cannot work them out. They have arguments and criticisms, haggling and nagging, and so you know where love goes. They have been developing weeds.

Where are the roses? They have not been nourished. We find out that we have been building up a life of resentment and resistance in our very homes and love should be in our home. I say this money problem is one thing we have to get rid of, this poverty consciousness. "I only have so much." Do you know you have everything; you have all the real riches of life? Would you trade greed for happiness? Would you trade money for happiness? What is all the money in the world worth, if you are going to be miserable? We must have a certain amount of happiness.

This reminds me of a little lady who wanted to spend her time with children and she said, "You know, if I could just take care of children, why, I would be the happiest person in the world."

I said, "Well, take care of children."

She said, "I am looking for a job and as soon as I get one I am going to stay with it." And she did, and she stayed for a couple of years at no pay. One day she was telling how happy she was and she just bubbled over when she talked about it.

Working just for money is not enough. There is an old saying that has meant a lot to me. "If you lose all of your money, you have lost a little; if you lose your health, you have lost a lot; but if you lose your peace of mind, you have lost everything."

One of my patients came in the other morning and said she had been cleaning the kitchen. She had washed down the whole kitchen that morning and painted it in the afternoon.

I asked, "Aren't you tired?"

She replied, "I am a little tired, but I have never been so happy in my life. My husband appreciates everything I do so much."

Appreciation is a wonderful thing. Do we have enough of these good things in our lives? I look at what greed, poverty consciousness, jealousy, hatred, and anger do to the stomach and to the glands, and then I say you will have to get rid of those bad things.

You know, they say that death is the last enemy to overcome. Well, let us look at this thing called death. You are all going to die someday. Everyone experiences the loss of a loved one at some time in his life, but there is no use living death before you pass away. There are people who are living death long before their time to die. It is like the girl who told me at one time that she was "just dying to get well."

Let us live to get well. We are using the negative processes to get well; but, you know, I had to look to the philosophy of a child to get me out of that feeling. I lost my beloved first wife when our son David was about a year and a half old. One day David and I took a ride down Wilshire Boulevard. Suddenly David said; "Mommy's dead, isn't she?" I was startled for a moment. Just why did he bring this out? No one had discussed it with him, at least I had not heard anyone discuss it with him. I thought as long as he had asked the question, I had better answer it.

I said: "Well, mommy isn't dead, exactly. Mommy has gone to another land."

"What does this land look like?" he asked.

I had never been so questioned quite so much; in fact, I looked at death as a finality, done, finished. David was, by his questions, forcing me to go a bit further in my reasoning on the subject of death.

I said, "David, I do not know what that land looks like. I have never been there. . . but I do know that we are all going there some day and we will all be together there."

Then he asked, "Can't you tell me what this land looks like?" And I said, "No, all I can say, David, is this land must be of the hands of God."

"What do the hands of God look like?" The child was not stopping. I could only answer, "Well, David, I cannot tell you that either. I have not seen the hands of God. I can only see his works, and everything is so wonderful that we must recognize that everything has been made by the hands of God. Someone must take care of the fallen sparrow. Every lily of the valley has been painted white. Someone must be taking care of that. . . and someone must be taking care of things in this other land."

He said: "Well, if mommy is in the hands of God, then she is in good hands, isn't she?" A child has given me a great philosophy!

You are going to have to decide whether it is in good hands or not. And for us to be in mourning, pining away over some loss, lonesome, feeling sorry for ourselves, is just a sign that we are looking for sympathy. This is a hard fact to face, is it not? You must recognize that your loss is of the flesh only; you have been attached to flesh and not to spirit; you have not been attached to any real philosophy of life.

You must let go; you must be free. Freedom is the greatest thing in life. If you cannot have your freedom, you are not even married; did you know that?

You cannot be married unless you are free. When I say that, I do mean that if you are a slave to your husband you are not married. You should be married in appreciation; you should be loved with complete freedom; you certainly are not together if you are not working together. If you cannot be trusted, then you are unworthy, this freedom that I speak of is mental freedom. . .and if you do not have mental freedom, it is impossible for you to have a good glandular condition.

Marriage should not drive you to go within yourself and become a hermit within yourself. Marriage should bring you complete expression of all your emotions, desires, and ideals. We find that there are many expressions which cannot be completed within ourselves, we need someone else to share what we have to give. There is no one you should be able to share as well with, as the one to whom you are married.

Marriage should be a release for real living. It should absolutely give you all the expression you have ever dreamed of or have ever thought of, in your mind.

To be cramped in any expression while you are married only brings on resentment and resistance. This, in itself, lowers the vitality of love and the sharing ability between the two.

The aging process comes over some people after they are married, only because they do not have the proper outlet of expression. They are hard on themselves because what they really do want, would perhaps hurt the other person. When we withhold our expressions, we are not completely honest with one another. We find that we cannot uplift the other person and this forces that person to feel inferior.

Oftentimes, a marriage is consummated and kept only through duty, or through the belief that it is the correct religious thing to do, or because the family does not believe in divorce. Certainly these people are not clean and clear in sharing the very finest within themselves, with one another. In order to live well, we must live for the highest good of man, for the higher good in each other. If we are not working for the higher good of man, and those who are the closest to us, we certainly should get to the bottom of the trouble. Freedom is what everyone is searching for, even though he be married.

In many cases, this lack of freedom can be dispelled when love takes its place. Love can heal; it is the most soothing balm we have to take care of our many negative attitudes. These negative attitudes, however, are not always brought into the open where we can see them. If they can be brought out in expressions of some kind so that the other person could know them, we find we can get together and getting together is very important to all marriages; you cannot live alone and be married.

The ovaries in women and the testicles and the orchic glands in men are exactly alike. These are the glands of procreation, the glands of new life. The next generation is dependent upon the ovaries and the orchic glands for its existence. They are in a different position, but they have exactly the same function, these glands produce from the men, spermatozoon, and from the women the ovarian follicle. The relation between the two, when they combine, produce all the male faculties and all the female faculties of the father and the mother and the wife and husband. When these two cells are joined together, a new body is born. We must recognize that; in these two cells we have the power to form in a new body. There had to be thought, the mind force, and then the word which becomes flesh. We live out a lot of our mother and father faculties from a physical standpoint. There are many things I do not like and the only reason I do not like them is because of the development I have had through heritage. It becomes necessary for us, in some cases, to overcome certain heritage in order to fulfill our own life.

The ovaries and the uterus in women control menstruation. Actually the blood of menstruation comes from the uterus, and this is what brings down the ovarian follicle. There is a little tube leading from the ovary right to the uterus and we find that the ovarian follicle goes into the uterus, the blood carries it down and we have what we call a "period" or a "cycle." We call this a cycle because we are subject to the natural, universal law. The moon makes a cycle every twenty-eight days and the moon controls the liquids of the earth.

The moon controls the tides and the waters of the earth. Women's menstruation periods are affected by the moon cycle. We find that women who menstruate before the full moon usually have pains, aches, and complaints. You can change that menstrual date through fasting and right living. . .and avoid having a difficult time with your period.

We also find that twenty-eight days may be normal for one person and others will menstruate every two weeks; but this may cause anemia. We then have to take care of the bloodstream. There may be one bad ovary and an indication of this is if one menstruation period is without pain and the next is painful; each period is controlled by one ovary. Usually when we speak of an ovarian condition, we have a little cyst on the ovary. This is like a little boil, a little infection; and this we clear up by various methods.

The toxic condition of the liver can depend upon several things; the lack of exercise, no hobby, working at one job all the time, sitting down all day long. There could be many reasons. It can be from a lack of proper relations between man and wife at home, whether it be with their money, their sleeping conditions, or their sexual communions. All these things can cause congestion in the different glands.

Men are dependent upon the bloodstream but they are also dependent upon balance in their life. I mentioned hobbies; there is no man who can work at a mental job all day and come home and do a mental job at night. He must have a hobby. You cannot be well sexually—you cannot be well physically—unless you have a hobby. Most of us are wearing out certain brain cells doing our job, but there are a lot of talented brain cells which are not being touched and which we can use in hobbies or in an avocation. Relax those brain cells, which are being used all day, and allow them to recuperate for a time. Why strain your body through excess concentration when tired?

I received a letter: "My problem concerns my husband and me!" As you know, a doctor is a father confessor and he gets about everything, as exemplified here:

"My husband is an honest man." . . . Is that enough? Do you want someone who is just honest walking around in your home? Honesty does not *make* a man, or woman either—there is something more.

"He is a hard worker." ...Is an honest man a hard worker? Is a hard worker enough?

"BUT, he is domineering and overbearing!"...Is she a nagger? Is she causing the trouble? Well, I do not know, but this is her side of the story anyway.

"He leaves me no freedom."...What did I tell you about freedom? "He is neither moral nor otherwise; he forces himself, his views and his will on me at all times and is very powerful physically and mentally; he is not at all spiritual; I live a suppressed life for he blocks my every move in every direction." ...What would you expect to get out of that woman? What do you expect to get out of that man? Are they married? *No!* They are hanging together.

"He has an ungovernable temper. His physical passion overwhelms him. He abuses me, becomes violent and cruel—even vicious and beastly. He is very coarse and humiliates me continually before my son, my friends, and everyone. Is there a remedy? What should my attitude be? How can I regain poise, my self-respect, and peace of mind?" . . . These are the things people want.

In getting married when we are young, we are overcome with passion; we are overcome with the flesh and our physical desires...but a real marriage is one made of heavenly thoughts and is made in a proper mental attitude. To just have a common interest of the mind maybe in music, art, some sport, or a certain peacefulness, is not enough.

If this peace is broken up by wrangling, nagging, by incompetency in making the other person feel good most of the time, we find that we are married in vain.

A person who gets married on the spur of the moment will probably find that he gets along well in about one percent of his life. There may be a time when we can appreciate music together, but that is one percent and only one! How about the other 99 percent that has to do with our money problems, the kind of home we are going to have—or the number of children we want?

Some people do not like children. I have seen homes where the wife would be better off working than staying at home taking care of her children.

Any housekeeper could take care of her children better. There are some women who just are not good mothers. . .and there are some men who are not good fathers. We make it so easy to get married and so difficult to get a divorce—while it should be just the opposite. We should make it very difficult to get married and easier to get a divorce!

Attitude is so important!...And let me tell you that our *attitude* is our *altitude*! It really is one and the same. Attitude is indeed altitude when you remember that your altitude is the level in life you are seeking. Your attitude is the level in life that you walk.

I have a story that shows what I mean concerning this level in life: There was once a prince who was looking for a cure for his troubles. After many doctors had failed him, he decided to find a man in his country whom he had heard was doing a lot of good for people. This man (a country doctor) looked over the prince and then suggested he wear the shirt of a *happy* man!

...So the prince commissioned representatives to find and obtain the shirt of a happy man. After a long period of time they returned and when the prince asked where the shirt was, they replied: "We found the happy man—but—he has no shirt!"

This only demonstrates that many times our philosophy is built up on physical things in life and when some of the physical things are taken away from us, our very life is taken also. This was demonstrated so destructively in the last depression when so many who had lost their money, committed suicide. Their entire world was founded on a cash basis and when that was gone, their world crumbled into nothingness.

Thoughts are things! We have to be careful that we are not possessed by things...or allow these things to possess us. We have to be careful that we are not victims of this world—rather than masters.

We must be careful of the suggestions that come to us. We cannot allow everything to come into our world and destroy us. We must know that beauty on the outside starts from the inside. That the beauty of our face very definitely comes from the spirit within. A beautiful soul will make over any face; we cannot see an ugly face when we recognize the light that is pouring from within.

There is always the possibility that even well-meaning people can make a suggestion that will burn you up, irritate you—or suggest something to you that causes your memory to grow and develop. The glandular memory process you develop in this manner also develops disease (dis-ease) in the body and in the glandular system. The glands are the greatest drivers we have in the body. They are also the greatest soothers—but they follow the suggestions in your body and you *must* get them in order first.

I live in Pasadena—and there is a story told about the Colorado St. Bridge, known as 'Suicide Bridge." They have put up a big fence to keep people from jumping off. According to this story, a young man was driving across. He stopped his car, got out, and started to climb the fence so he could jump off the bridge. A police car came along at that time and stopped. The officer got out of the car, climbed the fence after the boy, pulled him by the leg and said: "Say, son, come on down and let's talk this over." The boy did come down and after they talked for a half hour...they both jumped off!

When we analyze suicides, we find the people were misfits. They were not financially happy—love affairs were not working out—they had misunderstandings; they discovered their health was poor; they were riding on frayed nerves—or something was radically wrong in their lives, whether it was physical, mental, or spiritual.

When they desire to end it all, they are trying to get away from themselves. They are unable to stand their own nervous body. They know there *is* a peace of mind and of soul and in seeking this are not able to place it in their own body, which is broken down through this mental attitude.

When we have this lack of understanding, it is difficult to see that good *can* happen through changes. It is God who takes care of us through all changes in life. Most of us, when we are sick, want to get away— run away. We want to leave ourselves. Many of these runaway complexes in people are due to a lack of proper glandular balance.

In jumping off, let us make sure that we are jumping in the right direction. We all have the privilege of jumping, but there is only one right way.

We hear it said every day that we are just as young as our glands. This is construed to mean that we must take care of our glands in order to have youth expressed in our body. This sprightliness, vigor, and energy we find in the body, is not all found in the glands. We may have an aging person, but this aging is not always just in the glands. We may have a lack of certain chemical elements. We find that iron and oxygen are the two frisky horses in the body that keep us quite young. . .and sodium is of the minerals that is so necessary to keep us youthful. These things are found in the blood.

We find that life and the efficiency of our body begins to decrease on a poor diet and we must keep proper minerals flowing through our bloodstream, through what we eat.

There is no life in pills, no success in drugs, no beauty in lipstick, and there is no rejuvenation of gland life that is permanent in our glands alone. Youth and efficiency are found definitely in the blood. Bad foods can leave us helpless . . .and when we produce an acid condition in our body through bad combinations of foods, we find that acidity develops out of this kind of living and then our real trouble starts.

Acidity is the grim reaper in life and doctors and undertakers have just too much to do, because of our wrong eating habits. We turn ourselves into dust and ashes—even in our youth—and we continue to look for some spectacular gland food that can carry us on thru life. But, after all, it is in our living habits that our youth or our age is produced. We are just as young as our thoughts and we are just as old as our fears. We are as young as our blood and as old as the mineral balance found in our foods!

The blood, as it passes through the body, is picking up hormones that are secreted from different glands. These hormones have a job to do—just like every other secretion or fluid in our body. These glandular hormones are mixed with the blood, bathing material that goes over every cell in our body. Every cell in the body depends on the hormones that come from these glands.

We quicken our expression and our action; for example, to preserve our self—jumping away from an automobile, with the secretions that come from the adrenal glands. The person who is frustrated may produce hot flashes to the head, through thoughts and by what is happening in the thyroid gland. When these glandular secretions are not working into the bloodstream in the proper proportion, we develop a good many complications.

All the systems of the body are so connected that we cannot do without any of them. Every system, whether it be the circulatory system, the nerve system, the gland system, the elimination system, the thinking system, are all connected one with the other. If one is not expressing properly, every other system will feel this and be hampered accordingly.

It is so necessary to get our diet habits in order, for the blood carries the hormones and the hormones carry our thoughts; all work in harmony one with the other. The blood stream cannot have material in it that is made from coffee and doughnuts, chocolate, mineral oil; if we expect the finest results in every part of our body. Even working in reverse, we find that the best thoughts cannot be produced in the body, if the physical body is not right. We cannot expect a good physical body to express itself properly if the mind and the thoughts are not right. We cannot expect joy to be expressed in our body when we are living on coffee and doughnuts.

It may sound strange to you, but you picked this body when you came into this world. It is for you to accept experiences and to find the philosophy by which you can be the master. You are only on one road and your goal should be to master the problems you meet. What you may consider a fault may be a blessing. You must accept these faults and bless them and find the good in them and go on.

Let us get our whole body straightened out, get a rejuvenation of spirit, and a rejuvenation of the mind, and then the physical things, which take care of the glands, will be very easy. The rest of the body supports the glands. Your blood supports the gland activities, and if you stimulate this gland activity, you will have to expect an underactivity later because that is the law of compensation. When the heart has been overworked through running or jumping you will find that it needs a rest and in that rest period the heart will beat ten, fifteen times a minute less than it normally does. The whole body works that way.

Another thing for us to think about is, that as we grow a little bit older, we go through a change in life, many people object to and do not want to go through this change in life, but it is not what we want to do, in the body, the body follows natural law. The physical body does not know what to do; it just follows the law of the universe. You give your body too much sunshine and it gets burned. You do not like the burn. Your mind was not touched by the sun. Your body is the thing that is touched by the laws of the universe and we follow these laws. When we reach the age between forty and fifty we go through the change of life. It is a physical change of life but due to the fact the physical body is directly united with the mind, you can also expect changes of the mind at that time. Most people only have the changes of the mind through the fact that they are losing the same activities of the body. We find that their alertness is lessened when they do not have the glandular supply with which to work. If we overwork our mind tiring it out, wondering, condemning, and trying to comprehend, then the mind, as well as the physical body, is broken down.

Let us realize that this physical body has a change to go through, a natural change. Women are not going to menstruate all their lives. Nature is interested in this menstrual period for procreational purposes and for the new generation and she gives us a body of perfection from twenty to forty for the next generation's use. Nothing is really taken away from us from the age of twenty, to the age of eighty, except what we see in our own mind.

Do not think for a minute that women are the only ones going thru changes. We have mean irritable men, just like we have women—because they, too, go through changes just like women. When we recognize that men are constituted much the same as women in their glandular structure, we realize that they also go through changes. Vitamin E is a wonderful vitamin to use during this time of physical change. It is necessary for you to get your diet worked out, set up a corrective exercise routine, and start thinking correctly.

There is one thing that we must realize; after this change of life we do not have the quick response or the muscular control of the body that we had before. The glands themselves give us the power to contact, to tense, to relax, and we find that the glandular activity is never as good after the change of life as it was before; physical endurance and physical activity are lessened.

We go through this change only to enter into a more mental plane of life, a higher realm. We should be able to develop a higher expression in life. Who is the man who has the greatest amount of wisdom? We do not find much wisdom in young people. We do not find it in the physically-minded person. We find it in the person who has had experience, and as we go into life of wisdom, we find that we do not need the physical body as we did when we were young. We do not chase streetcars and do the daring things in our mental life we did in our physical life. We must accept the fact that going into the mental plane of life is a blessing to us. This is just a process of life that we must go through. There are some who do not want to accept this change and start fighting it, and they live through a fight in the change of life rather than through a blessing. If we do not accept the good things that come to us, we are in a war with ourselves through lack of understanding. It is this war that keeps the glands in a turmoil. If your body is going to make a change, accept it naturally and do not interfere with the process of change.

The body can grow from a physical standpoint, until you are about forty years of age and after that it stops growing. We find the recuperative ability is not as fast, but our mind goes right on growing. In order to think, we have to accept thoughts, which travel ahead at the same rate of speed, whether we are at the age of eighty or twenty and so we find that we have to change our attitudes in life. We have to change our mental aggressiveness to fit our physical aggressiveness. Most of us still want to jump over a six-foot fence at the age of eighty like we did when we were twenty. We find that we can still do things mentally and spiritually at eighty that we did not even think of when we were twenty. So, we take out a new life entirely; as we get older it should be a life of wisdom, reminiscence, and joy.

The joy centers in the body are not physical and all the operations in the world cannot find the joy center. When we are able to find this joy center in our life and use and develop it, even in our younger years, the more we extend our glandular activity. Most of us ruin our glandular activity through our mental activity. If we are not fighting our self, we are fighting everyone else, and it is this fight in our life that is interfering with the proper activity of these glands.

Some women go through this change earlier in life than others and this is usually due to the fact that they did not start to menstruate until they were thirteen or even sixteen years of age. This is a sign that the ovaries are not as strong as they would be if they had started to menstruate at ten or eleven. The woman who has strong ovaries, and her inherent powers are from strong parents, will start to menstruate early and will not go through the change until later years.

Some college performed an experiment in which they were told that one half of them would be given a special three-day examination. Cards were handed out to the students and fifty percent of the cards were marked "no examination." The students were told that all would have three days off whether they were taking the examination or not. Those who received the "no examination" cards were then seated on one side of the room, the others on the other side of the room. A photographer snapped the expressions and you should have seen the different expressions on the faces of those who had three-day examinations to take and those who were allowed to go free. Another interesting experiment was performed when a group of people were told they were going to inherit $25,000. You ought to have seen the vitality and the vim and vigor of expressions on those faces. Yes, I can see you smiling, too.

I know a man who had a hundred thousand dollars and lost it all except ten thousand dollars. He was a poor man; he could hardly get along on just ten thousand dollars; he was used to having a hundred thousand to work with. Another man who never had more than ten dollars most of his life, inherited ten thousand dollars and he was as happy as he could possibly be. One was miserable with ten thousand dollars and the other was happy. Where do you stand? What, or how much, does it take to make you happy? That is something for you to think about. So we see that our attitude really is our altitude. It depends entirely upon how we see things.

Worry is one of the things that drains the body and the nervous system and we may drain all chemical elements out of the body through worrying. Most worry is useless anyway, as we find that what we have on our mind this week, to be concerned about, will be changed entirely next week. There is a difference between worrying and being concerned about something. Many of us are worrying and taking care of our problems mentally when we are not capable of taking care of the problem ourself in the first place.

We have to decide whether the attorney or the doctor is going to take care of us, or whether we are going to leave it to God. It is wise to take our problem to the proper authority to help us, but worrying does not help and is one of the greatest wearing-out processes we have to our nervous and glandular systems. Our companions can cause a breakdown of the glands or they can build them up. We find that it is necessary to pick out companions that make us feel good. Some people depress us; some cause high blood pressure; others make us feel very peaceful. It depends entirely upon the attitude we have with that person.

Telegrams can send your blood pressure soaring. What causes this? The secret of living life successfully is this: There are two things to change—the world and yourself. If you cannot change the world, then you must change yourself. Do not try to make someone change, for it cannot be done. You will merely put yourself in poor health trying to do it. A good plan for life is the following: "God grant me the serenity to accept things I cannot change, courage to change the things I can, and wisdom to know the difference."

Beauty operators know that when a woman has been drinking a lot of alcohol she cannot be given a permanent. You cannot maintain a permanent in your hair if you drink a lot of liquor. Liquor also affects the pituitary gland. In a drunkard the pituitary gland becomes depressed, smaller, and that person is—what is he, a beast or a brute or a laughing hyena? In other words he has lost his identity as a man or a woman. Did you know that vinegar destroys the red blood cells in the body, just the same as alcohol? It also has a bad effect on the glands. One pint of vinegar can destroy twenty percent, or one-fifth of the red blood cells in the bloodstream. Blood travels thirty feet every second. Do you realize that the blood goes through every organ and every tissue and bathes every cell in your body every hour? What you ate yesterday is in this blood and is expressing itself in your feelings and your appearance today. We see, therefore, the vital importance of the food we put into our system.

Just as we have taken the mental side and recognize that we must eliminate the thoughts that are bad for us, we now consider the physical side, our diet program. If we are going to change our thoughts we must also change our diet, so let us consider all the changes that should be made. There is a mental diet as well as a physical diet.

We know that many of the foods we have today are stimulating. A good example is the use of gasoline in an automobile; it runs the automobile but it does not do any particular good. White sugar does the same thing in the human body. We have a pet name for coffee "Norwegian gasoline." It just makes your body run but there is no good there. Everything that goes into the body should nourish it. Avoid preservatives, condiments, heavily salted foods, pickled pigs' feet, and all of the different varieties of stomach ache on the market shelf.

Did you ever really look at a bottle of tomato ketchup? It has so little tomato in it, it is unbelievable. Examine a box of jello; it is only eight percent gelatin and eighty-five percent white sugar. The balance is artificial flavoring and coloring. White sugar is the greatest arthritis producer known and the greatest acid producer. White sugar works the glands harder and breaks them down quicker than anything else known. White sugar and white flour are two of the worst curses you can put into the body. If you want good health and youthful glands you had better abandon this type of food.

In cooking it is necessary to preserve the natural minerals in the food. We do not want to give our body things which are broken down or preserved through the cooking processes. We want to keep all of the chemical and mineral elements it is possible to retain. Refined wheat is devoid of the germ of wheat which is found on the outside covering. Vitamin B and Vitamin E are two of the specific vitamins which are necessary for the glands and these vitamins are contained in wheat germ.

Wheat cannot grow without the wheat germ. People are today eating only the inside of the wheat with the result that the glands and the heart are deteriorating, and then the doctor prescribes wheat germ or Vitamin E for the glands and the heart. Why not eat the whole wheat to begin with?

Vitamin E is strictly a gland food and is called the anti-sterility vitamin. Some women cannot give birth to children because they do not have the proper vitamin control in the body and the ovarian follicles cannot be produced and developed in the ovaries because of a lack of Vitamin E. That same condition exists in men. The most specific vitamin you can take in mental disorders, ovarian trouble, orchic disorders, sexual disorders, is Vitamin E.

The next highest vitamin is Vitamin B and it should be taken in complex form. Vitamin B complex is specifically for the nerves, and as the glands and the nerves work interrelatedly, Vitamin B is important. So let us take both Vitamin B and E for both the glands and the nervous system.

Vitamin B cannot be held in the body properly unless it is imbedded in a little fat or oil, and this oil is lecithin. You receive no good from Vitamin B unless you take lecithin with it and the greatest amount of lecithin is found in egg yolk. Some people must be careful, however, because egg yolk will cause liver disturbances. Almonds contain a great deal of lecithin, and black bass or smoked black cod are very high in lecithin.

Commercially we get lecithin from soybeans. There is a little green soybean called Miller's soybeans and when it is put in liquid form it is heavy and thick and extremely high in lecithin. The lecithin we buy in capsule form commercially comes from soybeans. It would be necessary to consume ten or fifteen pounds of soybeans in order to get the amount of lecithin we need in the body from day to day. If we do not use the egg yolk to get lecithin, then we should buy lecithin capsules in the health food store. Many of us are lacking lecithin and lecithin is one of the main fats necessary to rebuild the nervous system. Anyone who has arthritis must have lecithin. Lecithin has been burned out of our body whenever we have sore joints, neuritis, rheumatism, and arthritis. Lecithin is burned out by use and our bodies are being burned to ashes in our modern living processes, burned out when we are living a life of deterioration.

Here is a gland food cocktail that we give those patients who need a glandular rejuvenation and pick-up:

One tablespoonful wheat germ
Two tablespoonsful rice polishings
One egg yolk

Mix the above in grape juice or black cherry juice. These two juices are high in iron, which is necessary for the glands. You do not need a full glass of black cherry juice as it is concentrated. So if you want to add water or pineapple juice, you may. You may even put the mixture in pineapple juice, if you wish.

Iodine is very necessary so we can add one half-teaspoon of kelp powder or one half-teaspoon of Nova Scotia dulce to the foregoing recipe. This dulce is a seaweed that comes from the Eastern Coast and grows under a great deal more resistance than the kelp does in the warmer water of our Pacific Coast. The Atlantic Coast kelp is purple in color and is very high in manganese which is a specific element needed by the brain and nerve tissues. Pineapple juice and onions are very high in iodine and we need iodine for thyroid troubles. The best source of iodine, however, is clam juice. Mix clam juice with tomato juice or make a broth out of it as this is one way of getting soluble iodine into the body quickly. Make sure that you get unsalted clam juice.

A lot of people who want to gain or lose weight wonder what is wrong with their glands. A layer of fat tissue on the hip is caused by an ovarian disturbance, did you know that? We find a little bit of fat on the upper part of the hip and that is from the pituitary gland. When the pituitary gland is affected the wrists are small and the arms get larger and larger as they reach the shoulder. The same condition is reflected in the legs; the ankles will be small and the legs get larger and larger as they progress to the hips. This indicates a pituitary gland condition.

The secret of this whole thing is that we do not treat just one gland in order to get well. We work for good health generally and when we work for good health, the glands normalize themselves. We will not have to worry about any particular gland. Sometimes we have to take spot reducing or spot exercises for different parts of the body to get good blood circulating in there to carry away the fat. Beware of trying to reduce with thyroid, pituitary, or any of these different gland substances. Leave this to the doctor. There are all kinds of gland foods known to the profession but they should be taken only under a doctor's supervision. A short time ago it was discovered that doctors were giving reducing tablets that had dinitrophenol in it and many cases of blindness developed from people using this weight reducing remedy. This is a drug and you must be careful how you use drugs because most drugs are producing serious complications. I say this most sincerely because there definitely is a program of right living you could adhere to and be well. People are not getting well by using drugs. They are going on the same diseased way, receiving only temporary relief from these drugs, and doing nothing to eliminate the basic cause of the disease.

If you want to go on living on coffee and doughnuts and using aspirin to get rid of your headaches, it is all right; we have a well-equipped profession to take care of that. The automat system in New York, where you put your nickel in the slot for a cup of coffee or a hamburger, are now putting out a little package of Alka Seltzer with each meal. They know that you are going to need it. There is a restaurant in Hollywood, which has a sign reading, "We serve baking soda after every meal." That is one place you need it. I do not go in there!

If you come to me as a patient and you are living in a restaurant I cannot help you get well. There are over two million people eating three times a day in restaurants in this country and I am sure this figure compares favorably with the sickness we have.

I do not want to give you misinformation, but I show you the exaggerated condition so that we can readily see that poor, misguided eating and living habits are hurting us and can ruin our lives. We are definitely fooling ourselves.

In glandular disturbances there is one bath that will do more toward getting rid of menstrual disorders and rejuvenating and getting rid of trouble in the prostate gland than any other treatment and that is the sitz bath. This bath is not only for the glands but for the whole body. This sitz bath is one of the finest things I know of for driving the blood into the internal abdominal organs and that is where these sex glands are. The sitz bath is taken in the following way: Put about five inches of cold water in the bathtub (cold water is live water, while hot water is dead water). Sitting in the tub, keep the feet out of the water. Put the feet on a little stool, eight inches high, so that the legs and feet are out of the water. Cold water drives the blood from the surface inwardly and there is a surge of blood that goes into the internal organs, and this is what we need and want. This bath should be taken every day for three months for about five to ten minutes. It should be taken between periods if you are using it for menstrual cramps. Take the bath for three months and then drop it for a while and come back to it later. It can lose its effect, but if you let it go for a while and then come back to it again it regains its effect.

The basis for transforming the body and for a cure is good blood, free from all toxic material. Keep the bowels clean. Eat only good live food, which contains chemicals necessary to rejuvenate every organ in the body. Calcium, silicon, iodine, manganese, all the different chemicals we need, are found in natural foods.

You are made from dust and dust is a chemical. Get the necessary chemicals into the body and you can build the proper organs. Get that blood stream right and circulating where it is needed. If you are congesting these different organs, especially the sex organs, through your thinking, bad food, and poor eating habits over a period of years, start now to do some constructive work. Rather than wait for years for a healing to come about, because nature is slow, we can add to the natural principles by using this sitz bath and driving the blood into these organs.

You need not shock your system by using cold water the first day; start out by using some warm water and each day getting the water cooler and cooler. Soon you will be able to take it; we take things through resistance. You must learn to resist cold water in order to take cold water. You cannot resist the sun, wind, draft, or the rain until you get out in it. If we are going to sit on a pillow all our life, then we are going to need a pillow all our life. You get strong by doing the things that make you strong. Get in and use the muscles and the body and the mind. The law is that we must find the balance; if we overuse we break down; if we underuse, we are starving and underdeveloped. The same thing applies to the glands as every gland in the body follows these two principles; we either break them down through overusing or starving and not using at all, you cannot be well either way.

The third thing in getting well is rest. Rest cures. Doctors do not cure.

An exercise I consider very important is the figure eight exercise. A little lady came to me who had spent more than two years trying to get rid of a tumor of the uterus. She vowed that she would not have an operation. I worked very hard but we did not get rid of that tumor. I recognized the fact that we were not getting anywhere with this lady, so I asked her to take up hula dancing, and do you know that in six months' time the tumor was gone.

In the South Seas they do not have these tumors. When we stop and think how we walk down the street with packages or a purse in our arms and never use the abdomen or swing the hips at all, we see that we do not have any activity in the abdomen. You are meant to use that abdomen but we are not doing so. The figure eight exercise is very similar to the hula dance. Imagine a figure eight on the floor, stand in the middle of the figure and move the hips to make the figure eight. This moves the lower spine and loosens it up, stretches the abdominal muscles, puts these organs in better tone, and it is one of the finest things known for menstrual cramps or prostate disturbances. Use this exercise for five minutes, a couple of times a day. Please do not try this in front of a big department store or someplace where they will run you in; but you must have some closet in your house where nobody can see you! Let us do a little exercise.

I use iridiagnosis in my work and I find many people with arthritis and spinal troubles. In taking pictures of the spine through the X-rays, I find many of the cases of arthritis are missed by the average doctor because they will not show up on the X-ray. The iris of the eye would show me that arthritis was present so I wanted to get this on the X-rays. Every time take a picture now of the spine, I take one sideways, a lateral view, and do you know I find that arthritis is inside of the spine, next to the abdomen. The arthritis seems to be on the inside of the spine, next to the abdomen before it is on the outside, and that is why so many doctors are missing it with the average X-ray pictures.

Out of hundreds of spinal pictures I have taken, there are no cases of arthritis in the neck that did not start in the lower back. I am convinced that we must take care of that lower back much better. When you stop and think about it, the material for the glands, that are fed by the nerves, come from the spine. They must have a free flow, and in the lower back the nerves reach out to the liver, the ovaries, and to every gland in the abdomen. That is why it is so necessary to keep this part of the body limber.

Dancing makes a good hobby, especially the rhumba and the samba. My dancing teacher told me at one time that dancing is just like going to a good psychiatrist; it helps you mentally to express yourself, and to get all the exercise necessary to balance it.

I have developed a small exercise machine that embodies all of the movements I have been talking about. We call it the wigglefier. This machine works and exercises all the organs in the lower spine and abdominal regions and we use it in our reducing programs and to overcome tumors. One overweight lady lost three inches around her waist and hips in one month by using the "wigglefier" three minutes a day. The use of this machine stimulates circulation in the lower abdominal regions and this acts as a wonderful stimulant to the glands.

So many people say the mind was the beginning. Yes, mind is the beginning. Peace and war both start in the hearts of men and women. Love starts in the heart. That beautiful activity of gland force, the peacefulness and the ease that we seek in our heart, is found in the glands also. We find that dis-ease is not always in the form of some abnormal discharge or a breaking out. Dis-ease can come from tension. We keep the blood from circulating properly through tension, and the time comes that toxic material settles in these tension centers and organs, and in the thyroid gland particularly, it is said in the good book, "woe be unto you who has a stiff neck." When people want to get even with you, they get you in the neck. When I treat people and adjust their necks I can feel their money troubles, their husband troubles, their love troubles, their financial problems; they are all in the neck, so you have to keep the neck limber.

The thyroid gland is found in the neck and it is the most abused gland of all. Occupations that we follow today are very hard on the thyroid gland. Getting everything out by five o'clock! We are whistle listeners, clock watchers; we are always under pressure, get up, get out, serve, get it done, do not miss, make a promise, crawl to get there. We always have time to meet, time is in our consciousness. These things are all hard on the thyroid gland.

Here is an exercise that will help the thyroid gland tremendously, but first you must have a straight neck. You can have a straight neck by not using a pillow at night. Do not use a pillow. The next thing is to correct our posture by properly balancing the body. For example, if we have one short leg, we would not walk as though we had a short leg but would balance our self by stretching the upper part of the spine and pulling the neck up straight. You may develop two curves in the spine due to a short leg. The same thing happens when we wear high heels or when we have a large abdomen, bay windows, some people call them. When we have an extended abdomen we produce a curve in the lower back and we cannot walk straight as this causes a person to lean backwards. This forces the neck forward and the head back, and so what have we? We produce pressure on the thyroid gland.

We may also develop a curve in the upper part of the back when we have an extreme curve in the lower back. This is a compensatory curve in the upper part of our back, particularly in our neck, developed from the curve in our lower back. This curve in the upper back is what develops the extended Adam's apple and is caused by pressures on the thyroid gland. These pressures will interfere with the proper blood supply into the thyroid gland, and no matter how brilliantly you think, how good the food is that you eat, or how much iodine there is in your food, you will squeeze that gland to the extent that you will not get the blood there that is so necessary for the proper functioning of this thyroid gland.

Pressure symptoms must be considered in the body, as a tense-free body is necessary for good health and we should not have these abnormal curves. A prolapsus in the abdomen interferes with proper circulation to other organs. We must have a free-working body, one of good posture, with normal and natural curves. Tenseness hampers good circulation.

So, we see that posture is very important because the glands are affected by our posture. We should, therefore, strive to eliminate any abnormal curve in the spine. One exercise for this is to stand up against the wall, place the hands in the lower part of the back. If you can get your hands between your back and the wall, you have just that much of a curve to eliminate. When you have a big curve in the back you walk with an extreme jar to the whole body, but when you eliminate this curve you will find that you will walk with a nice, easy step. A curve in the back pushes some of the vital organs out of the proper position and subjects them to undue pressure. So, we see the importance of having a straight back.

We can see now that we start with ourselves. We start with a process of giving to a better life, a higher life. Can you accept the one fact that there is a better life for you? Can you reach for a better life? You can only reach this higher life through a good mental and physical body. Your glands play a big part in this. The best glandular cocktail that I could give to you is the fact that you are all possible gods. This is difficult for you to accept though, is it not? Some of you are born lowly and you remain that way. You are afraid to step out of the old; afraid to walk in a new pattern. There is nothing to fear but fear itself. Love yourself out of this and see the beauty in life; see the beauty that is in a rose and you will see the beauty that is in yourself. Allow the Godly things to exist in you. Church will mean nothing to you unless you are a walking church. If you cannot see the beauty that is within you, then who else will see it? Let your light shine; do not dim, diffuse, or hide it under a bushel. When we allow light to shine we draw unto ourselves all that is good. We must learn to mold, to give up. We should learn to forget, forgive, and go on to better things. These are all Godly processes of right living.

When we speak about love, Luther Burbank at one time said that he would never hire a man who did not love flowers. That is something for us to think about. Edwin Booth once considered that there was a king in every person and that he acted to kings. Are you powerful enough within yourself to assume the role of a king? Do you think there is enough beauty in you to be a rose? Would you dare walk like a queen? We must seek beauty and the nicest things in one another. He, who has conquered himself, has done more than he who has conquered a whole city.

## OTHER BOOKLETS BY DR. JENSEN

1. HOW TO ENJOY BETTER HEALTH FROM NATURAL REMEDIES

2. HOW TO RELAX AND RELIEVE TENSION

3. HOW TO REVITALIZE YOUR GLANDS

4. A NEW SLANT ON HEALTH AND BEAUTY—SLANT BOARD

5. A HEALTH PATTERN TO LIVE BY

6. HOW TO BUILD A BETTER BODY FROM YOUR KITCHEN

7. HOW THE BREATH OF LIVE SUSTAINS YOU

8. PHYSICAL, MENTAL AND SPIRITUAL BALANCE

9. DEVELOPING INWARD CALM

10. THE NEED FOR A NEW ATTITUDE

11. THE HEART OF CIRCULATORY SYSTEM

12. THREE STEPS TO THE HIGHER LIFE (Part I)

13. THREE STEPS TO THE HIGHER LIFE (Part II)

14. THREE STEPS TO THE HIGHER LIFE (Part III)

15. HEALTH FOR OUR CHILDREN

16. SPECIAL FOODS FOR SPECIAL NEEDS

17. LETS BEGIN AT THE BEGINNING

18. YOUR LOVE LIFE

19. INTESTINAL DISORDERS & FASTING & ELIMINATIVE DIETS

20. VOL. I — SECRETS I CAN SHARE WITH YOU

21. VOL. 11 — MORE SECRETS I CAN SHARE WITH YOU

## MEET THE ORIGINAL AUTHOR

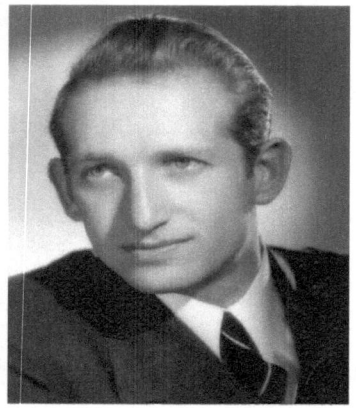

(From the back of the booklet)

Bernard Jensen, D.C, N.D., Nutritionist of Los Angeles, Calif. Born in Stockton, Calif, in 1908.

Possessing a convincing philosophy that would credit much older practitioners, Bernard Jensen, D.C, Lecturer and Teacher of Right Living, acquired from the beginning of his studies the vision "that Nature does all the healing." He believes doctors can only work with natural laws. His work is sane, up-to-date, practical, and teaches a balanced "how-to-live" regime.

At only 18, Dr. Jensen began studies with the West Coast Chiropractic College, Oakland, Calif. At 21 he began his practice of chiropractic in that city and has been practicing that science ever since. Widely traveled, he has been honored with post-graduate degrees from the National College in Chicago and the American School of Naturopathy, New York. He studied methods of the Battle Creek Sanitarium, of Tilden's School of Fasting in Denver. At an early age he was teaching his "How-to-live" methods to professional groups.

For 50 years. Dr. Jensen has led a most strenuous life, lecturing, radio broadcasting, and directing his own health center in Escondido, California.

His current plans include Radio and TV guest appearances, a nationwide tour, and more contributions to Iridology and color, with new works planned in both areas. Dr. Jensen's The Science and Practice of Iridology has brought him international acclaim and is currently being translated into Spanish. Nine more books are in various stages of production, including his spiritual masterpiece. Arise and Shine, and color book.

# HIDDEN VALLEY HEALTH RANCH

## <u>Comfortable Accommodations</u>

The accommodations are gaily decorated and furnished with every comfort—restful beds, spacious closets, and individually controlled heat. Each room will assure you a pleasant stay and a full night's sleep every night. Every attempt is made to make you as comfortable as possible. Accommodations are available at various rates to suit you.

Experience a new way of life, a non-demanding, relaxing, revitalizing way of living. Nestled in rolling country and continually blessed by pure fresh air, the ranch stretches over 200 acres of nature's artistry.

Your Hidden Valley vacation, or weekend, may well become a recurring part of your recreational plans. It is here that we make the best use of nature...organically grown food, exercise, pure water, and the right mental attitude all contribute to a vacation of unsurpassed value. Sun worshippers will enjoy the pool area or a leisurely walk around the ranch and hills can satisfy the desires of strollers, walkers, or hardy hikers.

## ABOUT THE AUTHOR

Jon Jensen, Iridologist, CMH, has been involved in holistic health for over 30 years with experience in Iridology, nutrition, and personal self-development. Jon started taking classes in Iridology and nutrition from his grandfather, the late Dr. Bernard Jensen, in 1980. Dr. Bernard Jensen is generally regarded throughout North America as the forefather of Iridology. Jon filled numerous roles over the years and participated in his grandfather's many classes and projects. Jon was involved in research for his grandfather's books, helping to pioneer a new way of iris analysis using the computer, and assisting with seminars.

In 1995 Jon stayed by his grandfather's side after Dr. Bernard Jensen became paralyzed from the waist down from a car accident. Jon was an integral part of his grandfather's plan to walk again, treating the whole person; body, mind, and spirit, and being a part of every aspect of what the doctors called a "Miracle"—as his grandfather walked again on his own.

After his grandfather's recovery, Jon shifted his attention to additional training by taking classes with some of the prominent leaders in the fields of Sclerology with Dr. Leonard Mehlmauer, Rayid (emotional iridology) with Denny Johnson, European based integrated iridology with Dr. Ellen Tart-Jensen as well as animal iridology with Dr. Mercedes Colburn. Jon attended Kalos© classes with Dr. Valerie Seeman-Gersch learning about Transformational Healing methods.

Jon was President of the Escondido Chapter of Chamber Toastmasters and enjoys speaking to groups.

Jon wrote an article for The Price-Pottenger Nutrition Foundation Journal on Animal Iridology/Nutrition. Jon has given presentations at: Holistic Health Fairs/Expo's, Herb Shops, and Health Food Stores.

Jon is currently Executive Director at the "Live Pure Kids" foundation in Arizona. Jon works closely with Gavin Tucker the President/Founder, and Jackie Morales, Vice President. The foundations Mission Statement: To educate our next generation through a disease prevention, mindfulness yoga, organic health, and wellness public school lifestyle program that empowers all children to encompass and build a strong foundation of equanimity with increased academic and behavior rigor starting from within—out. Live Pure Kids is dedicated to educating the next generation on how to live a healthy lifestyle by encompassing a holistic approach to life through balancing the mind, body, and spirit: www.livepurekids.com.

Jon recently published a nutrition book called, "A Simple Guide to Healthy Living" and it is available for purchase on Amazon.

For more information Jon can be found at www.jensenholistichealth.com www.bernardjensen.org

www.ingramcontent.com/pod-product-compliance
Lightning Source LLC
Chambersburg PA
CBHW021244280526
45784CB00005B/2236